THE JOURNEY THROUGH MENOPAUSE

"A Comprehensive Guide to Empower Women through the Phases of Change"

By

Linda A. Ivey

THANK YOU FOR CHOOSING US.

We Appreciate Your Kind Support And We Hope You Got Something Out Of It.

If You Enjoy This Book, It Will Be Great To Leave a **Review On Amazon** . It Means a Lot To Us.

Copyright ©y by Linda A. Ivey 2023.

Contents

Introduction:

A woman's menopause is a normal and unavoidable stage of life that signals the end of her reproductive years and the start of a new one. The timing of this shift, often known as "the change," can vary greatly from person to person and normally takes place between the ages of 45 and 55. Physical, mental, and hormonal changes occur during this period, which can have a significant impact on a woman's well-being and general quality of life.

Understanding menopause entails understanding the intricate interplay of hormonal changes and their wide-ranging impacts on a woman's body and psyche in addition to recognizing the cessation of menstruation. Menopause is a common experience for women, yet each woman goes through it in her way.

Why Menopause Is Important:

There is no way to overstate how crucial it is to comprehend menopause. A woman goes through this transition at a pivotal point in her life, when she must deal with not only bodily changes but also emotional and psychological difficulties. Menopause affects a person's relationships, self-esteem, and general health in addition to them.

With knowledge and tips to assist women in managing this shift with assurance and grace, this thorough book strives to shed light on the many aspects of menopause. In this section, we'll examine the mental and physical changes that come with menopause, go through the available treatments, examine how nutrition and exercise fit into this stage of life, and look at ways to keep close connections.

Additionally, we'll examine the psychological effects of menopause, including mood swings, anxiety, and sadness, and provide tips for coping with these difficulties. We will also look into natural treatments and complementary therapies for symptom relief, with a focus on a holistic approach to health.

This manual is intended to be a helpful tool whether you are approaching menopause, already experiencing it, or supporting someone who is. Our mission is to empower women by giving them the information and resources they require to view menopause as a fresh start, a period of self-discovery, and a chance to enjoy life to the fullest.

So let's set out on this trip together, striving not only to comprehend menopause but also to celebrate the courage and fortitude that each woman who goes through this crucial life change possesses.

Whispers of change

"The Story of Eleanor"

In the heart of a quaint town nestled between rolling hills and ancient oak trees, lived a woman named Eleanor. She was a mosaic of strength, wisdom, and grace, a beloved presence in the community who had weathered the seasons of life with resilience. Little did Eleanor know that a new season was silently approaching—one that would bring about profound transformations, both within her and in the fabric of her daily existence.

As the winds of change began to whisper through the leaves, Eleanor found herself at the threshold of menopause. The signs were subtle at first, like the delicate rustle of leaves before a storm. An occasional night of restlessness, a fleeting warmth that seemed to emanate from within, and a quiet introspection that colored her thoughts. Eleanor, always attuned to the rhythms of nature, sensed that something was shifting, a dance of hormones orchestrating a symphony of change deep within her being.

Her journey through menopause unfolded like the turning of pages in a well-worn book. The initial chapters brought with them the mystery of physical transformations—subtle yet undeniable. Eleanor felt the ebb and flow of hormones, like the rhythmic pulse of the river that meandered through the heart of the town. There were moments of warmth, akin to the gentle glow of sunrise, and nights where the moonlit sky mirrored the cool calmness that settled over her.

Emotionally, it was a tapestry woven with threads of introspection and self-discovery. Eleanor found herself revisiting the chapters of her life, reminiscing about the joys and challenges that had shaped her. The once vibrant hues of youth were now blended with the richer, more nuanced shades of maturity. Each emotion, a stroke on the canvas of her experience, painted a portrait of a woman embracing the fullness of her existence.

The community around Eleanor, much like the diverse flora that adorned the landscape, played an integral role in her menopausal tale. Friends and confidantes, some ahead on the same path, offered camaraderie and shared insights. The women in the town, like a sisterhood of seasons, whispered stories of their own menopausal journeys, fostering a sense of unity in navigating the unknown. Eleanor's family, the cornerstone of her life, observed the changes with an unwavering love. They became allies in this journey, adapting to the evolving cadence of their matriarch's needs. It was a time of mutual understanding, where conversations deepened, and bonds strengthened, creating a foundation of support as solid as the roots of the ancient oaks.

Yet, amidst the changes, Eleanor realized that menopause was not just an individual journey; it was a collective experience, a silent narrative woven into the very fabric of womanhood. It was a testament to the resilience and adaptability imprinted in the DNA of generations of women who had walked this path before her. As the pages turned, Eleanor embraced the metamorphosis with a sense of gratitude and acceptance. Menopause was not a culmination but a continuation—a bridge to a new chapter of life that held promises of wisdom, empowerment, and a deeper connection to the essence of womanhood.

And so, in the heart of that quaint town, Eleanor's menopausal journey became a narrative not just of change but of transformation—a story whispered by the winds of time, a story echoed in the rustling leaves, and a story that would resonate in the hearts of women who, like Eleanor, discovered the beauty in embracing the whispers of change.

Chapter 1

The Menopausal Transition

- **Defining Menopause and Perimenopause**

Menopause and perimenopause are two periods of a woman's reproductive cycle that are separate but closely connected. To successfully traverse this transitional time, it is crucial to comprehend these terminology and the changes they involve.

The Period Just Before Menopause

Perimenopause, often known as the "menopausal transition," is the period before menopause. It usually begins a few years before the actual onset of menopause and includes the period when a woman's body gradually starts to transition from its reproductive phase to its post-reproductive phase. Perimenopause is characterized by a variety of hormonal and physical changes, and it may continue anywhere from a few years to over ten years.

Among the main indicators of perimenopause are:

- Menstrual periods may become erratic, with fluctuations in cycle duration and adjustments to flow. This is often among the first indications of perimenopause.
- Hormone Level Fluctuations: As hormone levels, notably those of estrogen and progesterone, begin to change, several symptoms, including hot flashes, mood swings, and vaginal dryness, begin to appear.

- Many women go through perimenopause with menopausal

symptoms, however, the severity might vary. Hot flashes, nocturnal sweats, mood swings, insomnia, and changes in sexual drive are typical symptoms.

- Fertility Decline: During perimenopause, fertility steadily decreases. Although it is still possible, the chance of conception declines as a woman moves through this stage.

It's crucial to acknowledge perimenopause as a distinct and significant period in a woman's life. Each person experiences perimenopause differently, with different symptoms and difficulties. Women may handle the changes more successfully by being aware of this time and seeking assistance and knowledge.

The last menstrual cycle is called menopause.

When a woman approaches menopause, her last menstrual cycle has occurred. This is a physiologic change that normally happens between the ages of 40 and 50, however, individual circumstances may affect the precise date. A lady is formally diagnosed with menopause after she has gone 12 months without having her period.

Menopause's key features include:

Menopause signifies the end of a woman's natural capacity to procreate. The ovaries stop producing eggs after menopause, which ends fertility.

1. **Hormonal Changes:** Oestrogen and progesterone levels, in particular, sharply decline after menopause. Numerous physical and emotional problems might be caused by these hormone changes.

2. **Menopausal Symptoms**: While certain perimenopausal symptoms may continue throughout menopause, others may lessen or eventually go away. Hot flashes, mood swings, vaginal dryness, and changes in bone density are typical symptoms.

3. Despite being a momentous life event, menopause does not signal the end of a woman's life or her ability to serve. Instead, it marks the start of a new stage that may bring with it more freedom and chances for personal development.

4. Menopause and perimenopause are normal life stages for women. Women may be empowered to negotiate these changes with grace and confidence by being aware of them, accepting them, and looking for support and knowledgeable advice. The chapters

that follow will go into further detail on the physiological, psychological, and emotional elements of these stages and provide tips for dealing with the particular difficulties they present.

- **Common Age of Onset**

The average age of onset for perimenopause and menopause varies for every woman, although there are some basic recommendations for when these stages commonly occur:

Perimenopause: Perimenopause often occurs in a woman's 40s, although it may begin as early as her late 30s. The precise age of onset varies greatly across people. It often lasts many years before menopause. Menstrual irregularities, hormonal changes, and the development of menopausal symptoms are all frequent perimenopausal symptoms.

Menopause is formally diagnosed after a woman has gone 12 months without having a menstrual cycle. In the United States, menopause begins at the age of 51. Women may enter menopause at any age, ranging from their late 40s to their mid-50s. Menopause may be influenced by factors such as heredity, lifestyle, and general health.

It is crucial to note that, although these age ranges serve as a broad guideline, there is no one-size-fits-all solution, and individual experiences may differ. Some women may experience perimenopause and menopause sooner or later than expected. Furthermore, early menopause (before the age of 40) and premature menopause (before the age of 35) are conceivable, with separate reasons and implications.

- **Menopausal Symptoms Overview**

The intensity and length of menopausal symptoms might fluctuate greatly from one woman to the next. The hormonal changes that take place during perimenopause and menopause, especially the decrease in estrogen levels, are the main cause of these symptoms. Here is a list of typical menopausal symptoms, albeit not all women will experience them:

1. Hot flashes, often referred to as hot flashes, are rapid, strong sensations of heat that generally start in the chest and extend to the face and neck. Hot flashes and night sweats are two different conditions. Hot flashes known as night sweats happen when you're sleeping and can cause sleep patterns to be disturbed.

2. **Irritability and Mood Swings:** Hormonal changes may cause irritability, mood swings, and emotional ups and downs. During this period, some women could exhibit signs of worry and despair.

3. **Vaginal Changes**: As estrogen levels fall, the lining of the vagina may become thinner and drier, causing pain and dryness in the vagina as well as a higher risk of autism.

4. **Changes in Libido:** During perimenopause and menopause, many women report lower libido, which is often brought on by hormonal changes, pain from physical changes, or psychological issues.

5. Changes in hormone levels might cause sleep patterns to be disturbed.

Common concerns include difficulty sleeping and frequent nighttime awakenings.

6. **Cognitive abnormalities**: Some women claim that menopause causes memory loss, concentration problems, and cognitive abnormalities. This is also known as "menopausal brain fog."

7. **Weight Gain:** Modifications in the metabolism and hormonal equilibrium may make it simpler to put on weight, especially around the abdomen.

8. **Osteoporosis and Bone Health**: As estrogen levels fall, bone density may be impacted, raising the risk of osteoporosis and fractures.

9. **Cardiovascular Changes:** Oestrogen protects the cardiovascular system, thus when it declines after menopause, the risk of heart disease may rise.

10. **Breast Tenderness:** Some women may feel changes in the density of their breast tissue as well as breast tenderness.

11. Joint Pain: Hormonal imbalances may lead to joint pain and stiffness.

12. Headaches: During perimenopause and menopause, some women may have more frequent or severe headaches.

It's crucial to remember that not all women will have all of these symptoms, and some women may suffer just a few or minor symptoms throughout their relatively painless journey through perimenopause and menopause. However, there are several therapy choices and lifestyle changes that may help control and ease these difficulties for individuals who do have moderate to severe symptoms.

Chapter 2

Physical Changes

- ### Hot Flashes and Night Sweats

Hot flashes, sometimes called hot flashes, are defined by abrupt, strong heat waves that usually originate in the chest and spread to the neck and face. These episodes can range in duration from a few seconds to several minutes, and they frequently come with an increased heart rate and perspiration. Aim for 150 minutes or more per week of moderate-to-intense exercise. They can happen at any time of day, hot flashes are most frequently linked to the evening (night sweats).

Hot Flashes That Don't Go Away at Night

In essence, night sweats are hot flashes that happen while you're sleeping, and they can be very bothersome. When you have night sweats, your sleep patterns may be disturbed and you may wake up drenched in perspiration. Fatigue and a lowered general sense of well-being may result from this.

Handling Night Sweats and Hot Flashes:

Although dealing with hot flashes and night sweats can be difficult, there are ways to assist control and get rid of these symptoms:

Lifestyle Modifications: Even small lifestyle adjustments can have a significant impact. To assist in controlling your body temperature, wear layers of clothing made of natural, permeable materials. Steer clear of alcohol, caffeine, and hot, spicy foods as these might cause heat flashes. At night, keep the room at a cool temperature.

Frequent Exercise: Regular physical activity can assist in controlling body temperature and enhance sleep. Aim for 150 minutes or more per week of moderate-to-intense exercise.

Reducing Stress: Anxiety and stress can make hot flashes worse. These symptoms may be managed with the aid of stress-reduction strategies including yoga, mindfulness, and deep breathing.

Hormone Replacement Therapy (HRT): This treatment option may be available to women who have severe and incapacitating hot flashes. Hormone replacement therapy (HRT) replaces the hormones lost during menopause, especially estrogen.

Phytoestrogens: Including foods high in phytoestrogens in their diet helps some women who suffer from hot flashes. These plant-based chemicals, which are included in soy and flaxseed diets, may have a role in hormone regulation.

Prescription Drugs: A healthcare professional may prescribe specific prescription drugs to treat severe and ongoing hot flashes. Serotonin-norepinephrine reuptake inhibitors (SNRIs) and selective serotonin reuptake inhibitors (SSRIs) are two examples of these drugs.

- Weight Gain and Metabolism

Women face particular difficulties navigating this life-changing stage because menopause frequently causes changes in weight and metabolism. Women can take charge of their health management by being aware of the causes of weight increase and taking preventative action.

Elements That Lead to Weight Gain:

1. **Hormonal Changes:** The distribution of body fat may be impacted by the menopausal drop in estrogen levels. Abdominal fat accumulation is common in women and is linked to an increased risk of several health problems.

2. **Metabolic Slowdown:** As we age, our metabolisms naturally slow down, which makes gaining weight easier. Menopause-related hormonal changes may make this slowing worse.

3. **Loss of muscular Mass:** Ageing and a drop in exercise can cause a person's muscular mass to decline. Loss of muscle can lead to weight gain since muscle burns more calories at rest than fat does.

4. **Factors related to lifestyle:** Modifications in eating patterns and physical activity levels, for example, might cause weight increase after menopause.

Controlling Weight in the Menopause:

- **Frequent Exercise:** Keeping up a healthy weight and promoting general well-being require regular physical activity. Mix up your regimen by including strength training, flexibility, and cardio workouts.

- **Dietary Balance:** Prioritise eating a diet full of fruits, vegetables, whole grains, lean meats, and other nutrients. Limit your intake of processed foods, sweets, and saturated fats, and pay attention to portion sizes.

- **Strength Training:** Including strength training activities in your program will help you maintain weight control, increase metabolism, and fend off muscle loss.

- **Hydration:** Getting enough water in your diet is important for your general health and can help you manage your weight by making you feel full and reducing overeating.
- **Handling Stress:** Prolonged stress has been linked to weight growth. To assist in controlling stress levels, try stress-reduction methods like yoga, deep breathing, or meditation.
- **Sufficient Sleep:** Give adequate, high-quality sleep priority. Hormones that control hunger can be upset by irregular sleep patterns, which can lead to weight gain.
- **Hormone Replacement Therapy (HRT):** If a woman's quality of life is being adversely affected by weight gain, hormone replacement therapy may be appropriate in certain situations. But before deciding to use

HRT, you should balance the advantages and disadvantages and speak with a healthcare professional.

- **A Positive Body Image to Adopt:**
- Weight and body composition changes are normal during menopause, which is a period of transition. Instead of concentrating only on the number on the scale, it's critical to consider your general health and well-being. A happier and more satisfying menopausal journey can be achieved by adopting a positive body image and engaging in self-compassion exercises.

Personalized advice based on unique health needs and objectives can be obtained by speaking with a qualified dietician or healthcare professional. Keep in mind that each woman's menopausal experience is distinct, and overcoming this stage with resiliency and vigor requires a comprehensive approach to health and fitness.

- **Skin, Hair, and Nail Changes**

Along with visible changes to internal features, menopause also brings about noticeable changes to exterior features like nails, hair, and skin. Women may handle these changes with confidence and grace if they understand them and take a proactive approach to skincare and self-care.

Skin Modifications:

- **Dryness and Thinning:** Skin that is less elastic, moisturized, and produces less collagen may have decreased estrogen levels. Skin that is thinner and drier as a result may be more prone to wrinkles and fine lines.
- **Loss of Elasticity:** Skin becomes less elastic as a result of decreased collagen levels. The skin may look less tight and some areas of sagging may become more apparent.

- **Enhanced Sensitivity:** Some women may have more reactive and sensitive skin. Menopause can cause skin disorders like rosacea or eczema to flare up.

Changes in Hair:

- ❖ **Thinning and Loss: Changes** in hormone levels, especially a reduction in estrogen, can cause thinning and loss of hair. The texture of hair may also get finer.

- ❖ **Changes in Texture:** Hair may become drier or more prone to frizz due to changes in texture. The health of the scalp may be impacted by variations in sebum production.

- ❖ **Greying:** During menopause, the aging process naturally occurring in combination with hereditary factors might cause hair to turn grey.

Changes in Nails:

❖ **Brittlenes**s: The tendency for nails to break and become more brittle may occur. Decreased moisture levels and hormonal changes can have an impact on this.

❖ **Changes in development:** The pace of nail development may slow down, and dietary and blood flow modifications may have an impact on the general look of nails.

Tips for Hair and Skin Care:

• **Regular Moisturize:** To prevent dryness and preserve the flexibility of your skin, use a hydrating moisturizer. Make sure the skincare products you choose are suitable for your skin type.

- **Sun Protection**: To shield skin from the sun's damaging UV rays, which can hasten the aging process, use a broad-spectrum sunscreen with an SPF of at least thirty.

- **Gentle Cleaning:** Use cleansers that aren't too strong to remove natural oils from your skin. Steer clear of hot water as it may exacerbate dryness.

- **Hydrate from Within:** Make sure you get enough water each day to stay hydrated. Maintaining the health of your skin, hair, and nails requires adequate hydration.

- **Nutrient-Rich Diet**: Eat a well-balanced diet full of vitamins and minerals that are vital to the health of your skin, hair, and nails. Add meals high in omega-3 fatty acids and antioxidants.

- **Hair Care Procedures:** Apply gentle shampoos and conditioners based on the type of hair you have. Think about adding oils and nourishing hair masks to your regimen.

- **Frequent Trims**: Maintaining healthy hair and controlling the appearance of thinning can be achieved by regular hair trimming.

Maintain clipped and moisturized nails. To address brittleness, think about using moisturizing cuticle creams or nail strengtheners.

Recall that these changes are a normal aspect of aging, and accepting them as aspects of your beauty will help you approach menopause with confidence and strength.

- **Bone Health and Osteoporosis**

Navigating this part of the menopausal journey requires an understanding of the variables causing bone changes and the adoption of preventive strategies.

Affected Bone Health Factors During Menopause:

❖ **Decline of Oestrogen**: Oestrogen is essential for preserving bone density. Bone loss can quicken during menopause as estrogen levels drop.

❖ **Age-Related Bone Changes:** As people age, their bone density gradually decreases. Hormonal changes associated with menopause may make this normal process worse.

❖ **Absorption of Calcium and Vitamin D**: Hormonal fluctuations can impact the body's ability to absorb these two vital minerals for strong bones: calcium and vitamin D.

❖ **Physical inactivity:** Bone loss may be exacerbated by a sedentary lifestyle. Maintaining bone density requires strength training and weight-bearing activities.

❖ **Smoking and Drinking Too Much Alcohol**: These lifestyle choices might have a detrimental effect on bone health. Smoking and heavy alcohol use are associated with an increased risk of osteoporosis.

Proactive Steps to Maintain Bone Health:

* **Diet Rich in Calcium:** Make sure you're getting enough calcium from foods like dairy, almonds, leafy greens, and fortified meals. If your diet isn't providing enough calcium, think about taking supplements.

* **Vitamin D:** Natural sunlight contains vitamin D, which is necessary for the body to absorb calcium. Eat a diet high in foods high in vitamin D, and if necessary, think about taking supplements.

* Frequent Weight-Bearing Exercise: Take part in weight-bearing activities like strength training, walking, running,

or dancing. Bone density is increased and maintained by these exercises.

❖ **Give Up Smoking:** Giving up smoking can improve your general health, including the health of your bones. One of the risk factors for osteoporosis is smoking.

❖ **Limit Alcohol Intake:** For the best bone health, alcohol use should be moderated. Drinking too much alcohol might cause bone loss.

❖ **Bone Density Testing**: If you have risk factors for osteoporosis, talk to your healthcare practitioner about getting a bone density test. Proactive management becomes possible with early detection.

❖ **Hormone Replacement Therapy (HRT)**: To treat hormonal imbalances and promote bone health, hormone replacement therapy (HRT) may be advised for certain women. A healthcare professional should be consulted before deciding whether to pursue HRT, and the advantages and hazards to each patient's health should be taken into account.

Putting Strength in Your Bones for a Bold Future:

Proactively maintaining bone health both during and after menopause is an investment in your long-term health. Robust bones can be maintained by using a holistic strategy that incorporates a nutrient-rich diet, frequent exercise, and lifestyle modifications.

- **Cardiovascular Healths**

Hormonal changes during this era can affect many areas of heart health, thus lifestyle decisions and preventive care are crucial. Women are empowered to prioritize their heart health for a robust and vibrant future when they are aware of the links between menopause and cardiovascular health.

Menopause and Heart Health:

- **The Cardiovascular System is Protected by Oestrogen:** Oestrogen is a hormone that decreases throughout menopause. Its decrease may be linked to modifications in cholesterol levels and blood vessel function.

- **Elevated Cardiovascular Risk:** Heart disease and stroke are among the cardiovascular disorders that are linked to an increased risk during the postmenopausal era. This risk is also increased by variables like age, family history, and lifestyle decisions.

- **Cholesterol Level Changes:** Menopause can cause a rise in low-density lipoprotein, or "bad" cholesterol, and a fall in high-density lipoprotein, or "good" cholesterol.

- **Blood Pressure Fluctuations:** During menopause, hormone fluctuations may have an impact on blood pressure regulation and result in elevated blood pressure.

Techniques for Maintaining Cardiovascular Health During Menopause

- ❖ **Heart-Healthy Diet:** Eating a diet high in fruits, vegetables, whole grains, lean meats, and healthy fats promotes cardiovascular health. Refined carbohydrates, salt, and saturated and trans fats must all be consumed in moderation.

- ❖ **Frequent Exercise:** Take part in strength and aerobic training frequently. By enhancing cardiovascular fitness and preserving a healthy weight, exercise promotes heart health.

- ❖ **Weight control:** Retaining a healthy weight lowers the chance of developing cardiovascular illnesses. It has a favorable effect on blood pressure, cholesterol, and heart health when combined with regular exercise.

- ❖ **Give Up Smoking:** One of the biggest risk factors for cardiovascular illnesses is smoking. One of the most effective strategies to enhance heart health is to give up smoking.

- ❖ **Limit Alcohol Intake:** While moderate alcohol use is typically seen as appropriate, excessive use might increase the risk of cardiovascular disease. If taken, it ought to be done so moderately.

- ❖ **Frequent Health Check-Ups:** Make an appointment with your doctor frequently to evaluate your cholesterol, blood pressure, and general cardiovascular health. Timely intervention is possible with early detection.

❖ Developing Your Heart for a Future of Health:

Putting cardiovascular health first during menopause is a comprehensive strategy that includes food choices, regular health checkups, and lifestyle decisions. Women who adopt heart-healthy behaviors can not only more easily manage the changes brought on by menopause, but they can also build the groundwork for a heart-healthy and active future.

Chapter 3

Emotional and Psychological Impact

- **Mood Swings and Irritability**

Managing Mood Swings and Irritability During Menopause: Finding Emotional Balance

Mood swings and irritability are regular companions on the menopausal trip, which are frequently ascribed to hormonal variations that characterize this transforming stage of a woman's life. Understanding these emotional upheavals and implementing appropriate coping methods can provide women with the tools they need to handle mood swings and irritation with grace and perseverance.

Understanding the Root Causes

47

1. Hormonal Changes: The fluctuation and fall of estrogen and progesterone is the major cause of mood swings and irritability throughout menopause. These hormonal changes have the potential to affect neurotransmitters in the brain, hence impacting mood regulation.
2. Sleep disruptions: Hormone changes can cause sleep disruptions, and insufficient sleep can increase mood swings and irritability.
3. Menopause is frequently associated with other life transitions, such as children leaving home, professional changes, or caring for aging parents. These pressures can exacerbate emotional turmoil.

Mood Swings and Irritability Management Strategies:

- Exercise regularly since it has been shown to improve mood and reduce stress. Walking, yoga, and swimming can all be extremely useful.

- practices for Stress Reduction: Incorporate stress-reduction practices into your daily life. Deep breathing, meditation, and mindfulness are all practices that can assist in managing stress and creating emotional equilibrium.
- Adequate Sleep: Make excellent sleep hygiene a priority. Establish a consistent sleep schedule, develop a calm nighttime ritual, and make sure your sleeping environment is restful.
- A well-balanced diet rich in fruits, vegetables, whole grains, and lean proteins is recommended. Nutrient-dense diets improve general health, including emotional well-being.
- Social Support: Create and keep a solid support network. Sharing your feelings with friends, family, or support groups can help to give understanding and emotional support.

- Mind-Body Practises: Look into mind-body practices like yoga or tai chi. These exercises benefit not only physical health but also emotional and mental well-being.
- Professional counseling or therapy can provide a secure environment in which to examine and treat emotional issues. Therapists can help you develop coping skills and methods for dealing with mood swings and irritation.

Self-Awareness and Compassion:

It is critical to recognize that mood swings and irritability are natural components of the menopausal transition. Women can negotiate these emotional shifts more easily if they engage in self-reflection and practice self-compassion. Acceptance of one's feelings, along with proactive measures toward emotional well-being, constitutes a comprehensive strategy for coping with mood swings throughout menopause.

- **Anxiety and Depression**

Understanding Menopausal Anxiety and Depression:

1. Hormonal Changes: The reduction in estrogen and progesterone levels during menopause can influence neurotransmitters in the brain, contributing to mood and emotional well-being changes.

2. Menopausal symptoms like hot flashes and night sweats can interrupt sleep patterns, and sleep problems are connected to mood disorders including anxiety and despair.

3. Menopause frequently corresponds with numerous life transitions, such as children leaving home or work changes.

These adjustments might cause stress and emotional difficulties.

4. Personal and Family History: A personal or family history of mental health disorders may impact an individual's vulnerability to anxiety and depression.
5. Holistic Emotional Well-Being Strategies:

6. If medicine is required, it may be prescribed to ease symptoms of anxiety or depression. This choice should be made with the help of a healthcare practitioner.

7. Regular Physical Activity: Regular physical activity has been shown to improve mood and mental well-being. Aim for a combination of aerobic and strength training workouts.

8. Adopt a nutrient-dense diet rich in fruits, vegetables, whole grains, lean proteins, and healthy fats. Certain nutrients are beneficial to mental wellness.

Techniques for Mindfulness and Relaxation:

❖ Incorporate mindfulness practices, meditation, deep breathing exercises, or yoga into your daily routine. These approaches can aid with stress management and emotional equilibrium.

❖ Adequate Sleep: Make excellent sleep hygiene a priority. Create a calming nighttime routine, make sure you have a comfortable sleeping environment, and address any sleep problems that may be contributing to your anxiety or sadness.

❖ Build a solid support network of friends, family, and support groups. Sharing your thoughts and feelings with trusted people can give emotional support.

❖ Hormone Replacement Therapy (HRT): Hormone replacement therapy (HRT) may be explored in some circumstances to correct hormonal imbalances that contribute to mood disorders. This choice should be taken with the help of a healthcare expert, after carefully assessing the risks and advantages.

❖ Personalized Well-Being Approach:

It is critical to recognize that each woman's menopausal experience is unique and that there is no one-size-fits-all answer to emotional issues. Addressing anxiety and depression during menopause requires a personalized and comprehensive strategy that takes into account individual health, lifestyle, and preferences.

- Cognitive Changes

Common Cognitive Alterations:

Menopausal women may have periodic forgetfulness or memory lapses, which are sometimes referred to as "menopausal brain fog." These lapses are often transient and might be related to hormonal imbalances.

- ❖ **Difficulty Concentrating:** During menopause, sustaining attention and concentration might be difficult. This might be due to hormonal changes, sleep disruptions, or increased stress.

❖ Word Retrieval Problems: Difficulties finding the proper words or forgetfulness in ordinary discussions might be symptoms of menopausal cognitive changes.

Factors Influencing Cognitive Changes:

❖ Oestrogen, a hormone that decreases after menopause, has been connected to cognitive processes. Changes in estrogen levels can affect neurotransmitters and cognitive functions.

❖ Menopausal symptoms such as hot flashes and nocturnal sweats can alter sleep patterns, adding to cognitive problems.

❖ Stress and Anxiety: Increased stress levels, which are frequently related to the many changes that occur during menopause, can have an impact on cognitive processes.

❖ Age-Related Factors: Cognitive changes accompany aging, and menopause might aggravate these effects.

Cognitive Well-Being Supportive Strategies:

❖ **Regular Exercise**: Physical activity has been demonstrated to improve cognitive performance. Aim for a mix of aerobic and strength training workouts.

❖ Adopt a nutrient-dense diet rich in omega-3 fatty acids, antioxidants, and other brain-supporting elements. Fish, nuts, fruits, and vegetables all help with cognitive wellness.

- ❖ **Adequate Sleep**: Make excellent sleep hygiene a priority. achieve a calm nighttime ritual and address any sleep problems to achieve a consistent sleep pattern.

- ❖ **Mental Stimulation:** Engage in mind-stimulating activities such as puzzles, reading, learning new skills, or pursuing hobbies. Mental stimulation helps with cognitive resilience.

- ❖ **Stress Reduction:** Use stress-reduction strategies such as mindfulness, meditation, or deep breathing exercises to reduce stress. Stress management improves cognitive functioning.

- ❖ **Maintain frequent health check-ups to assess general health, including**

issues that may impair cognitive well-being.

Accepting Cognitive Changes as a Natural Part of the Process:

It is critical to recognize cognitive alterations as a typical feature of the menopausal transition. Women can face these changes with self-compassion, knowing that they are just transitory and frequently improve over time. Adopting a comprehensive approach that incorporates physical, mental, and emotional well-being adds to a more enjoyable menopausal experience.

Chapter 4

Nutrition and Menopause

- **Dietary Recommendations**

Paying attention to food choices becomes essential as women navigate the transforming phase of menopause to improve general well-being and manage particular symptoms linked with this life change. The following food suggestions should be taken into account during menopause:

1. Foods Rich in Calcium:

Relevance: Women going through menopause are more likely to experience bone loss. A healthy diet rich in calcium promotes strong bones.

Sources: Almonds, dairy products, fortified meals, and leafy greens like broccoli and kale.

2. **Calcium (D)**

Significance: Crucial for absorbing calcium and maintaining bone health.

Sources include sunshine, fatty fish (mackerel, salmon), fortified meals, and supplements as needed.

3. **Fatty Acids Omega-3:**

Significance: Promotes heart health and might perhaps mitigate mood fluctuations.

Fish oil supplements, walnuts, chia seeds, flaxseeds, and fatty fish (trout, salmon) are some of the sources.

4. **Complete Grains:**

Importance: Supply fiber, vital nutrients, and long-lasting energy.

Quinoa, brown rice, barley, oats, and whole wheat are the sources.

5. Trim Proteins:

Significance: Encourages the health of muscles and aids in preserving a healthy weight.

Fish, poultry, lean meats, tofu, lentils, and plant-based proteins are some of the sources.

6. Foods High in Phytoestrogen:

Plant-based chemicals that mimic the actions of estrogen are important because they may help reduce menopausal symptoms.

Sources: whole grains, flaxseeds, sesame seeds, and soy products (edamame, tofu).

7. Vegetables and Fruits:

Important: High in fiber, vitamins, and antioxidants. promotes general health and might aid with weight management.

Variety: To guarantee a wide spectrum of nutrients, include a vibrant assortment of fruits and vegetables.

8. Stay Hydrated:

Significance: Aids in reducing symptoms such as hot flashes and promotes general well-being.

It is advised to stay hydrated by drinking lots of water all day long. Infused water and herbal teas can offer diversity.

9. Restrict Sugary and Processed Foods:

Importance: Cutting less on processed and sugary foods improves general health and helps with weight management.

Other Options: Select whole, unadulterated meals and, if necessary, use natural sweeteners.

10. Moderate Alcohol Intake with Caffeine:

Importance: Consuming excessive amounts of alcohol and caffeine can have negative effects on general health and cause sleep disruptions.

It is advised to consume in moderation and to think about cutting back, particularly right before bed.

11. Foods High in Iron:

Significance: Essential for preserving energy levels.

Lean meats, chicken, fish, lentils, and fortified cereals are some of the sources.

12. Magnesium

Significance: Encourages bone health and might ease symptoms such as sleeplessness.

Sources: Legumes, nuts, seeds, whole grains, and leafy green vegetables.

13. Vitamin B:

Significance: Critical to the generation of energy and general health.

Sources: Leafy green vegetables, dairy products, eggs, chicken, fish, and whole grains.

14. Tailored Method:

Take into account that everybody has different nutritional demands. Pre-existing diseases, prescription drugs, and individual preferences are a few examples of factors to take into account.

.

Extra Advice:

- **Meal Planning**: To promote general nutrition, plan balanced meals that include a variety of macronutrients (carbs, proteins, and fats).
- **Maintain a Regular Eating Schedule**: To maintain energy levels and stabilize blood sugar levels, try to eat at regular intervals.
- **Mindful Eating**: To encourage digestion and develop a positive relationship with food, engage in mindful eating.

- **Managing Weight and Metabolism**

1. A well-rounded diet:

Lean Proteins: To maintain muscular function and metabolism, give priority to lean protein sources like chicken, fish, tofu, and lentils.

Whole Grains: For long-lasting energy and fiber, choose whole grains like quinoa, brown rice, and oats.

Healthy Fats: For satiety and general well-being, include sources of healthy fats such as avocados, nuts, seeds, and olive oil.

Portion Control: To maintain calorie balance, pay attention to portion sizes.

2. Frequent Exercise:

Cardiovascular Exercise: To increase metabolism and promote heart health, regularly partake in cardiovascular exercises like brisk walking, cycling, or swimming.

Strength Training: Incorporate strength training activities to maintain and increase muscle mass, since this might have a favorable effect on metabolism.

Exercises for Flexibility: To improve general fitness, including flexibility exercises like yoga.

3. HRT, or hormone replacement therapy:

Take into consideration: Hormone replacement treatment (HRT) may be a viable alternative for certain women to control menopausal symptoms, such as changes in weight.

Consultation: To make well-informed judgments based on unique health issues, and discuss the possible advantages and hazards of HRT with healthcare specialists.

4. Intentional Consumption:

Awareness: Recognise signs of hunger and fullness. Eating with awareness can help you avoid overindulging and encourage a positive connection with food.

Slow Eating: Enjoy each mouthful of your food and take your time when eating. The body can now identify satiety cues thanks to this.

5. Stay Hydrated:

Water Intake: Drink enough water since sometimes hunger and thirst are the same thing. Water is good for your general health and might help you control your weight.

6. Quality of Sleep:

Setting priorities: Make sure you get enough good sleep. Sleep issues have the potential to affect metabolism and cause weight gain.

Establish a calming nighttime routine and make your surroundings sleep-friendly about sleep hygiene.

7. Managing Stress:

Impact of Stress: Prolonged stress can alter metabolism and lead to weight gain. Include stress-relieving pursuits like deep breathing, meditation, or hobbies.

Balance: Make an effort to have a balanced life that incorporates enjoyable activities as well as relaxation.

8. Regular Meal Times:

Routine: To assist metabolism and give steady energy throughout the day, set regular eating times.

9. Tailored Method:

Consultation: For individualized advice, speak with licensed dietitians or healthcare professionals. Take into account personal preferences, underlying medical issues, and health-related considerations.

10. Community Assistance:

Connect with Others: Participating in online or in-person supportive groups may offer inspiration, motivation, and a wealth of shared experiences.

11. Self-compassion and Acceptance:

Mentality: Adopt an optimistic outlook. Acknowledge that fluctuations in weight during menopause are an inherent aspect of this time of life, and that self-compassion is crucial.

During menopause, controlling weight and metabolism requires a mix of dietary decisions, exercise routines, and lifestyle practices. Women may negotiate this stage with resilience if they use an individualized, comprehensive strategy that supports both weight control and general well-being.

- **Supplements for Menopause**

1. Vitamin D and calcium:

Significance: Crucial for maintaining healthy bones, particularly around menopause when osteoporosis risk rises.

Supplementation: If food consumption is inadequate, calcium supplements including vitamin D are frequently advised.

2. Fatty Acids Omega-3:

Significance: Preserves cardiac health, mitigates mood fluctuations, and enhances general wellness.

Sources: Walnuts, flaxseeds, chia seeds, and fatty fish (mackerel, salmon). Fish oil and other omega-3 supplements may be taken into consideration.

3. B-Complex Vitamin:

Significance: B vitamins are involved in the generation of energy and the modulation of mood.

Sources: Leafy green vegetables, dairy products, eggs, chicken, fish, and whole grains. Insufficient food consumption may warrant the consideration of B-complex supplementation.

4. Magnesium

Importance: Promotes muscular and bone health and may help reduce symptoms like sleeplessness.

Sources: Legumes, nuts, seeds, whole grains, and leafy green vegetables. If dietary consumption of magnesium is insufficient, supplements may be of consideration.

5. Kyanite:

Contributes to blood clotting and bone health, which makes it important.

Broccoli, Brussels sprouts, and leafy green vegetables are the sources. Supplemental vitamin K may be taken into consideration, particularly for people with certain medical issues.

6. Vitamin E

Antioxidant qualities and the ability to reduce symptoms like hot flashes make it important.

Sources: Broccoli, spinach, nuts, and seeds. Supplements with vitamin E may be used on the advice of a healthcare professional.

7. Cohosh Black:

Herbal Supplement: Some women find that taking a herbal supplement called black cohosh helps to manage menopausal symptoms including mood swings and hot flashes.

Be cautious: Speak with medical professionals as each person's experience with the safety and effectiveness of herbal supplements may differ.

8. Isoflavones from soy:

Natural Estrogen-like Compounds: Because soy isoflavones have estrogen-like properties, they may help alleviate some menopausal symptoms.

Sources: Soybeans and tofu items made from soy. Supplements are to be used with caution and by medical advice.

9. Prebiotics:

Important: Promotes intestinal health, which affects general health.

Sources: probiotic supplements and fermented foods (yogurt, kefir, and sauerkraut).

10. CoQ10 or Coenzyme Q10:

Antioxidant qualities and the possibility to promote heart health make them important.

Sources: Whole grains, meat, and fish. Supplementing with CoQ10 may be worthwhile, especially for people who have cardiovascular issues.

11. Calcium:

Antioxidant qualities, which promote immunological health, are important.

Sources: Broccoli, bell peppers, berries, and citrus fruits. Supplemental vitamin C might be taken into consideration, particularly for people with dietary restrictions.

12. Iron:

Menopausal women may still require iron, especially if they are deficient in certain nutrients or experience excessive menstrual flow.

Be cautious: Speak with medical professionals since consuming too much iron may have negative consequences.

13. Dehydroepiandrosterone or DHEA:

Hormonal Precursor: As we age, our bodies produce less DHEA, a hormone that some women think can help maintain hormonal balance.

Caution: Due to possible hormonal effects and specific health issues, it is important to consult with healthcare specialists.

Crucial Points to Remember:

Personalized Advice: Speak with medical professionals to receive advice that is specific to your requirements, circumstances, and state of health.

Supplement Quality: Select reliable brands to ensure both safety and quality. The effectiveness of supplements varies, and they are not all made equal.

- **Flexibility and Balance Exercises**

1. Yoga

Benefits: Yoga incorporates balancing postures, stretches, and soft motions. It helps general well-being, increases flexibility, and encourages relaxation.

Pose: Incorporate stances such as the Warrior series, Tree Pose, Cat-Cow, and Downward Dog.

2. Chi Gong:

Benefits: Focusing on regulated motions, Tai Chi is a gentle, flowing martial art that enhances flexibility, balance, and calmness.

Tai Chi exercises include "Cloud Hands," "Grasp the Sparrow's Tail," and "Waving Hands Like Clouds."

3. Pilates

Benefits: Pilates emphasizes regulated movements, flexibility, and strength in the core. It can enhance general body awareness and posture.

Exercises: Perform Pilates movements such as the Saw, Leg Circles, and the Hundred.

4. Exercises for Stretching:

Benefits of regular stretching include increased joint range of motion, decreased muscular tension, and increased flexibility.

Areas of Focus: Focus on the main muscular groups in your body, such as your shoulders, back, hips, and legs.

5. Exercises for Balance:

Benefits: Since menopause may cause a loss in bone density, improving balance is essential for preventing falls.

Exercises: Perform basic balancing exercises such as the heel-to-toe walk, the stork posture, or standing on one leg.

6. Dancing

Benefits: Dancing is a lighthearted approach to enhance balance, flexibility, and coordination. It also has advantages for the cardiovascular system.

Styles: Think of dancing to your favorite music in salsa, ballroom, or even free-form.

7. Exercises using Stability Balls:

Benefits: Using a stability ball improves balance and stability by activating the core muscles.

Exercises: Try some seated leg lifts, stability ball planks, and stability ball squats.

8. Bands of Flexibility:

Benefits: Resistance bands offer mild resistance for strength training and can be used to increase flexibility.

Exercises: Use resistance bands to perform torso twists, arm stretches, and leg stretches.

9. Aerobics in Water:

Benefits: Resistance training in water promotes muscular strength and flexibility while lessening the strain on joints.

Exercises: Perform arm circles, leg lifts, and water walking in a pool.

10. Wrist stretches and ankle circles:

Benefits: Simple exercises that increase joint flexibility and mobility include wrist stretches and ankle circles.

Motions: Make circular motions with the ankles and softly extend and flex the wrists.

11. Exercises with Foam Rollers:

Benefits: Using a foam roller helps increase flexibility and relieve tense muscles.

Exercises: Move the foam roller over your back, thighs, and calves, among other main muscle groups.

Mind-Body Techniques:

Benefits: Mind-body techniques like deep breathing and meditation can improve general well-being, lower stress levels, and improve physical flexibility.

Practises: Make time each day for mindfulness and relaxation exercises.

Crucial Advice:

Consistency: For long-lasting effects, incorporate frequent flexibility and balancing exercises into your program.

Safety First: Take care to use good form to avoid being hurt. Before beginning a new fitness regimen, speak with your healthcare professionals about any ailments or health issues you may have.

Develop Gradually: Begin with workouts appropriate for your present level of fitness and progressively raise the time and intensity.

- **Staying Motivated**

1. Make sensible objectives:

Set reasonable and attainable fitness objectives. Divide more ambitious objectives into more achievable subgoals.

2. Look for Fun Things to Do:

Take part in physical activities and hobbies that you truly like. Whether it's yoga, hiking, or dance, picking pursuits you like will make them more likely to continue with you.

3. Vary Your Daily Schedule:

Make your exercise regimen interesting by varying it up. To keep yourself from getting bored, mix up your workouts by including cardio, weight training, and flexibility exercises.

4. Plan a Regular Exercise Schedule:

Establish a routine for your exercise. Make exercise a priority in your daily schedule and treat it as such.

5. Companhia:

To make working out more fun, attend a group exercise class or work out with a friend. Having a workout partner fosters accountability and mutual support.

6. Monitor Your Development:

To monitor your progress, utilize fitness apps or keep an exercise log. Observing progress over time may be quite inspiring.

7. Give Yourself a Treat:

Create a system of rewards for reaching fitness benchmarks. Reward yourself with something fun when you accomplish a goal to encourage good behavior.

8 Pay Attention to Your Feelings:

Keep an eye on your feelings after working out. Having more energy, feeling happier, and having better overall health can be strong incentives.

9. Assign New Tasks:

Continually add new difficulties to your exercise regimen. It can involve taking a different fitness class, working out harder, or learning a new yoga posture.

10. Establish a Helpful Environment:

Embrace a helpful atmosphere around you. Tell your loved ones or friends about your fitness objectives so they can support and empathize.

11. Show Off the Long-Term Gains:

Imagine the long-term advantages of consistent exercise: better health, more energy, and a higher standard of living both during and after menopause.

12. Pay Attention to Your Body:

Pay attention to what your body requires from you and modify your exercise regimen accordingly. Provide time for relaxation and make adjustments as necessary to guarantee a long-term strategy.

13. Make It Pleasurable:

Include things that will add enjoyment to your exercises, such as upbeat music, being outside, or experimenting with new fitness routines.

14. Take Part in Fitness Challenges:

Take part in fitness competitions or activities. Events such as virtual races, step challenges, and fitness classes have the potential to foster motivation and a sense of community.

15. Practise self-kindness and patience

Recognize that obstacles are a normal part of the trip and that improvement takes time. In your pursuit of fitness, use self-compassion and patience.

Chapter 5

Managing Menopausal Symptoms Naturally

- **Herbal Remedies**

For millennia, people have used herbal treatments to treat a variety of health issues, including menopausal symptoms. Although the effectiveness of these treatments varies from person to person, some women find that using herbal medicines helps with certain symptoms. It is essential to remember that using herbal treatments should be done with caution and after consulting your healthcare professional, particularly if you are taking medication or have underlying medical concerns. The following herbal therapies are often thought to be effective in relieving menopausal symptoms:

1. Cimicifuga racemosa, sometimes known as black cohosh:

Potential Advantages: Known to have the ability to reduce mood swings and hot flashes.

Black cohosh may affect liver function; thus, be cautious and consult your healthcare professional, especially if you have liver issues.

2. Trifolium pratense, or red clover:

Potential Advantages: Contains isoflavone-containing chemicals, which may help alleviate hot flashes.

Be cautious: People who have a history of blood clotting difficulties or hormone-sensitive diseases should speak with their doctors.

3. Angelica sinensis, or Dong Quai:

Potential Benefits: This traditional Chinese herb is said to help reduce hot flashes and regulate hormones.

Use caution when pregnant and speak with your doctor, especially if you have a blood-clotting problem.

4. Oenothera biennis, or evening primrose oil:

Benefits: Contains gamma-linolenic acid (GLA), which has the potential to relieve hot flashes and breast discomfort.

Carefully consider consulting your healthcare professionals, particularly if you are using blood-clotting drugs or have epilepsy.

5. Panax ginseng, or ginseng:

Potential Advantages: Adaptogenic herbs have the potential to reduce tiredness, elevate mood, and enhance general well-being.

Use caution while consuming large amounts, especially in people with high blood pressure.

6. Vistalia agnus-castus, or chasteberry:

Potential Advantages: May lessen symptoms like mood swings and breast discomfort and help control hormone levels.

Be cautious: Speak with medical professionals, particularly if you suffer from hormone-sensitive diseases.

7. Salvia officinalis, or sage:

Potential Advantages: Helps lessen nocturnal sweats and hot flushes.

Use caution while incorporating culinary sage into your diet. Consult your healthcare professional for advice on sage supplements.

8. Hypericum perforatum, or St. John's Wort:

Potential Benefits: Known for elevating mood, it might help reduce minor depression or mood fluctuations.

Use with caution since it interacts with many drugs; first, speak with your healthcare professional.

9. Lepidium meyenii, or maca root:

Potential Benefits: This adaptogenic herb is said to help regulate hormones, libido, and energy levels.

Be cautious: Speak with medical professionals, particularly if you have thyroid problems.

10. Lavandula angustifolia, or lavender oil:

Potential Benefits: Used in aromatherapy to ease symptoms associated with stress and encourage relaxation.

Use essential oils carefully; they should not be overused. Speak with your medical professionals, particularly if you have sensitivities or allergies.

11. Flaxseed

Potential Advantages: Contains lignans, which may aid in the control of night sweats and hot flashes.

Use caution while including flaxseed in your diet. If you have any problems that are sensitive to hormones, speak with your healthcare specialists.

Subfamily Ginkgoceae: Ginkgo Biloba

Potential Advantages: Some women get improvement from memory loss and other cognitive issues.

Carefully consider consulting your healthcare practitioner, particularly if you are using blood thinners.

Crucial Points to Remember:

Individual Responses Differ: Everybody reacts differently to herbal medicines in terms of their efficacy.

Speak with Healthcare Professionals: Speak with your medical professionals before using herbal medicines, particularly if you use a prescription or have pre-existing medical issues.

Quality Is Important To guarantee quality and safety, get your herbal supplements from reliable providers.

1. A well-rounded diet:

Make eating a nutrient-rich, well-balanced diet a priority to promote general health.

Add foods high in calcium for strong bones, foods high in heart-healthy omega-3 fatty acids, and a range of fruits and vegetables for antioxidants.

2. Consistent Exercise:

Exercises that include aerobic, strength, and flexibility training should be done.

To make fitness a lasting part of your routine, choose something you like doing.

3. Managing Stress:

Use stress-reduction strategies including mindfulness, deep breathing, and meditation.

Make self-care activities that make you happy and relaxed a priority.

4. Sufficient Sleep:

Create a cozy sleeping environment and stick to a regular sleep schedule.

Resolve sleep difficulties right away, and seek medical advice if necessary.

5. Hormone-Related Matters:

When thinking about hormone replacement treatment (HRT), talk to medical professionals about the advantages and disadvantages.

Regularly evaluate the effects of hormone therapy and make necessary adjustments based on your health.

6. Mind-Body Methodologies:

For overall well-being, include mind-body exercises like yoga, tai chi, or meditation.

These exercises help improve mental clarity, emotional equilibrium, and physical flexibility.

7. Social Networks:

Spend time with friends, and relatives, and/or join support groups to foster social ties.

Building a solid support system is beneficial to emotional health.

8. Stimulation of the Cognitive Process:

Take part in mentally stimulating activities like reading, doing puzzles, or picking up new skills.

To maintain cognitive health, keep your mind engaged.

9. Introspection and Gratitude:

Accept yourself and the changes that come with going through menopause.

Acknowledge the lessons learned from life's experiences and rejoice in your development.

10. Frequent Medical Exams:

Plan routine medical check-ups with your physicians to keep an eye on your general health.

Respond quickly to any health issues and work with medical specialists to create individualized health programs.

11. Drink plenty of water:

To promote general health and reduce symptoms like hot flashes, drink enough water.

Drink plenty of water and other hydrating liquids daily.

12. Managing Your Time:

Set priorities for your work and use your time wisely to avoid stress.

Keep your expectations in check and be aware of your energy levels.

13. Recreation and Leisure:

Make time for hobbies and leisure pursuits that make you happy and relaxed.

Take part in things that make you feel happy and fulfilled.

14. Frequent Health Examinations:

Follow recommendations for screenings for heart health, osteoporosis, and breast cancer.

Long-term health is influenced by preventative actions and early identification.

15. Welfare of the Emotions:

Openly acknowledge and communicate your feelings.

If you need help navigating emotional problems, get professional help.

16. Integration of Hormonal and Lifestyle Adjustments:

Collaborate with medical professionals to include lifestyle and hormonal changes.

Make sure any lifestyle adjustments support your overall health objectives.

17. Adaptability in Daily Life:

Be flexible and willing to modify procedures in response to evolving demands.

Accept adaptability in both short-term and long-term goals.

- **Acupuncture and Alternative Therapies**

The promise of acupuncture and other alternative treatments to alleviate menopausal symptoms has drawn interest. Although each person's reaction is unique, some ladies find these strategies helpful. It's crucial to remember that the efficacy of various treatments may vary based on a person's health, preferences, and the particular symptoms being treated. Here are some other strategies to think about:

1. Acupuncture

How It Works: To promote energy flow (qi) and restore balance, acupuncture involves inserting tiny needles into certain body locations.

Potential Advantages: Acupuncture has been reported by some women to lessen hot flashes, enhance sleep quality, and enhance general well-being.

Think about it: Look for a qualified and skilled acupuncturist. During the session, go over your health history and symptoms.

3. Feedback from biofeedback

How Biofeedback Works: To lower stress, biofeedback teaches users how to regulate physiological processes like heart rate and muscular tension.

Potential Advantages: May ease the symptoms, such as hot flashes, and encourage calm.

Take into account: Qualified therapists may assist people in learning self-regulation strategies.

4. Meditation and yoga:

Yoga: Blends breathing exercises, meditation, and physical postures. may increase general well-being, lessen stress, and increase flexibility.

Meditation: Stress management and relaxation are two benefits of mindful meditation.

Taking into account: Guided sessions or classes taught by knowledgeable teachers might be helpful.

5. Chiropractic Treatment:

How It Works: To enhance general health, chiropractic therapy targets the musculoskeletal system via spinal adjustments.

Potential Advantages: According to several women, receiving chiropractic therapy has enhanced their well-being and decreased suffering.

6. Use of aromatherapy:

How It Works: By applying or inhaling essential oils topically, aromatherapy employs them to enhance well-being.

Potential Advantages: Some women report alleviation from stress and sleeplessness symptoms.

Think about this: Select premium essential oils and abide by use recommendations.

7. Body-Mind Connections:

Tai Chi: Consists of deep breathing and fluid, leisurely motions. may improve flexibility, balance, and general health.

Qi Gong: Promotes energy flow and balance by combining breathing techniques, meditation, and movement.

Taking into account: Structured practice may be obtained via classes or guided sessions.

8. Hypnotherapy:

How It Works: To treat certain issues or symptoms, hypnotherapy uses concentrated attention and guided relaxation.

Possible Advantages: A few ladies report feeling less anxious and getting better sleep.

Think about it: Look for a licensed and skilled hypnotherapist.

9. Therapeutic Massage:

How It Works: To improve relaxation and lessen muscular tension, massage therapy manipulates soft tissues.

Potential Advantages: Could reduce stress and symptoms including muscular soreness.

Select massage providers that are qualified and licensed with caution.

10. The practice of reflexology

How It Works: To encourage relaxation and balance, reflexology includes applying pressure to certain areas on the hands, feet, or ears.

Potential Advantages: For some women, hot flashes and other symptoms are relieved.

Think about hiring a certified reflexologist for your sessions.

Crucial Points to Remember:

Tailored Approach: Reactions to non-traditional treatments may differ. Be open to experimenting with new strategies since what works for one individual may not work for another.

Qualified Practitioners: To guarantee safe and efficient treatment while seeking alternative therapies, choose practitioners with training and experience.

Chapter 6

Maintaining Sexual Health

- **Changes in Libido**

- **Hormonal Fluctuations**: A reduction in oestrogen and progesterone levels during menopause might affect a woman's libido. For optimal sexual health and vaginal lubrication, oestrogen is essential. Some women may have dry vagina and decreased arousal when levels drop, which might affect libido.

- **Physical Changes:** Discomfort during sexual activity may be attributed to the physiological changes brought on by menopause, such as modifications to genital tissue and decreased blood supply to the pelvic area. A decrease in sexual desire or a reluctance to participate in intimate activities might result from these physiologic changes.

- **mental and Psychological Factors:** Anxiety, weariness, and mood swings are just a few of the symptoms of menopause that may negatively affect one's mental health. These elements may influence changes in body image and self-perception, which in turn affects sexual confidence and desire. They may also interact with social views on ageing and sexuality.

- **Relationship Dynamics:** Modifications in libido during menopause may also have an impact on these dynamics. In order to handle the emotional and physical parts of intimacy at this stage, open communication with a partner becomes essential. A satisfying and happy sex life may be enhanced by understanding and supportive partners.

- **Coping Mechanisms**: One of the most important aspects of managing the effect of menopause on relationships is recognising and treating changes in desire. Consulting medical professionals or sex therapists may give information about possible therapies, including hormone therapy or lubricants, to alleviate physical pain and improve sexual enjoyment.

- **Rediscovering Intimacy**: Going through menopause may provide couples the chance to experiment with new, close-knit relationships. A deeper connection may be achieved by putting an emphasis on shared experiences, communication, and emotional closeness. A useful component of this rediscovery might also include investigating non-traditional forms of physical intimacy.

- **Self-Care and Body Positivity:** Managing libido fluctuations requires embracing self-care techniques and fostering body positivity. Maintaining a healthy diet, getting regular exercise, managing stress, and managing one's general health may all have a favourable impact on mood and energy levels, which may increase a person's desire for sex.

- **Seeking Professional Advice:** Consulting with medical professionals is crucial if libido fluctuations have a substantial negative influence on quality of life. Depending on the specifics of each case, hormone treatment, counselling, or other therapeutic measures could be suggested. Personalised and successful plans are ensured by transparent and sincere engagement with healthcare providers.

In summary, libido fluctuations during menopause are a complex phenomenon impacted by hormonal, physical, emotional, and interpersonal variables. Maintaining a happy and meaningful romantic relationship may be facilitated by navigating this period with empathy, communication, and a proactive commitment to self-care. Since each person's experience is different, getting help when required guarantees a comprehensive approach to wellbeing during the menopausal transition.

- **Vaginal Health**

1. Hormonal Shifts and Dry Vagina:

Recognizing Hormonal Shifts: Dry vagina and thinned vaginal walls might result from decreasing estrogen levels throughout menopause.

Effect on Lubrication: Decreased estrogen has an impact on the production of vaginal secretions, which increases sensitivity to irritation and causes pain during sexual activity.

2. Moisturisers and Lubricants:

Water-Based Lubricants: Water-based lubricants may relieve some of the initial pain experienced during sexual activity.

Vaginal Moisturisers: Using vaginal moisturizers regularly helps maintain comfort since they are designed to hydrate and rebuild the vaginal lining.

3. Options for Hormone Therapy:

Estrogen-Based Therapies: To treat the symptoms of vaginal dryness, doctors may give estrogen replacement therapy (HRT) in the form of pills, creams, or rings.

Consultation with Healthcare professionals: Discuss possible advantages and disadvantages of hormone treatment with healthcare professionals depending on your unique health situation before deciding to pursue it.

4. Exercises for the Pelvic Floor:

Kegel exercises: By strengthening the pelvic floor muscles, one may improve general pelvic health and vaginal tone.

The Secret Is Consistency: Pelvic floor exercises, when performed correctly and consistently, can improve sexual and bladder control.

5. Frequent Intercourse:

Increasing Blood Flow: Having frequent intercourse increases blood flow to the pelvic area, which benefits vaginal health.

Open discussion about any pain or changes in sexual function with a partner helps to build understanding and support.

6. Sufficient Hydration:

Water Intake: Maintaining proper hydration promotes mucous membrane hydration throughout the body, including the vaginal region, and is important for general health.

7. Mild Cleaning Methods:

Gentle Cleansers: For the external genital region, use gentle, fragrance-free cleansers. Steer clear of douching and strong soaps as they might upset the delicate balance of the vaginal environment.

Cotton Pants: To limit moisture retention and lower the chance of discomfort, choose breathable cotton pants.

8. Frequent Check-Ups for Gynaecology:

Annual Examinations: Make an appointment for routine gynecological examinations to keep an eye on the health of your vagina, screen for any problems, and talk to medical professionals about any symptoms.

Early Detection: Timely intervention and treatment of vaginal health disorders are made possible by early detection.

9. pH balance of the vagina

Keeping Things in Balance: To deter dangerous germs, the vagina naturally keeps its pH acidic. It is essential to sustain this natural balance and stay away from harsh products.

Probiotics: Consuming probiotic-rich foods or supplements may help keep the vaginal flora in a healthy state.

10. Taking Care of Vaginal Atrophy:

Symptoms: Several procedures may be used to treat vaginal atrophy, which is characterized by the weakening, drying out, and inflammation of the vaginal walls.

Topical Treatments: Medical professionals may administer topical estrogen pills or lotions to help treat symptoms.

11.   Interaction   with   Medical Professionals:

Be Open with Your Healthcare Providers: Share any worries or symptoms about vaginal health.

Customized Care: Medical professionals can provide suggestions that are specific to each patient's symptoms and medical history.

12. Mental Health and Wellness:

Emotional Health: Since stress and worry may affect vaginal health, be aware of how menopausal changes affect emotional and psychological well-being.

Holistic Approach: Stress reduction and self-care techniques are part of a holistic approach to wellbeing, which supports general vaginal health.

- Intimacy and Communication

1. Transparent and Truthful Communication

Establish a safe space where both parties may freely communicate their worries and ideas without fear of repercussions.

Frequent Check-Ins: Plan frequent check-ins to talk about your experiences, emotions, and any changes in closeness. Promote empathy and attentive listening.

2. Knowledge and comprehension:

Study Together: Learn about the physical changes that come with going through menopause. Patience and empathy may be developed by being aware of the difficulties.

Consult a Professional: To acquire knowledge about handling menopausal symptoms and their effect on intimacy, think about going to educational seminars or counseling sessions together.

3. Mutual Assist:

Menopause may cause emotional ups and downs, therefore emotional support is important. Providing one another with assistance when one is feeling vulnerable strengthens the emotional bond.

Shared duties: Work together to alleviate stresses and create a supportive atmosphere by sharing duties.

4. Flexibility in Personal Activities:

Together, explore novel kinds of intimacy that put comfort and enjoyment for both parties first. Be willing to explore new things that suit the interests of both parties.

Prioritise Emotional Connection: Give emotional connection priority, making sure that intimacy extends beyond physical actions to encompass emotional bonding and shared experiences.

5. Handling Modifications to the Body:

Collaborative Healthcare Approach: Attend doctor's visits jointly to talk about and manage menopausal physical changes.

Speak with Medical Professionals: Consult your healthcare professionals for advice on how to manage your symptoms, and work together to find possible solutions.

6. Individual Needs Sensitivity:

Respect Personal Boundaries: Be aware that comfort levels might differ from person to person. Be honest and respectful of one another's personal space and preferences.

Validation and Affirmation: To build emotional intimacy, provide validation and affirmations. Small acts of gratitude can create a happy, emotional environment.

7. Closeness Outside of the Bedroom:

Prioritise quality time spent together, even when it's not at personal times. Take part in things that help to build an emotional bond, such as walks, hobbies, or just spending time together in silence.

Surprise gestures: To create an atmosphere of closeness in daily life, surprise each other with kind acts that express your love and gratitude.

8. Spread Knowledge About Hormonal Shifts:

Gain a shared understanding of how menopause's hormonal shifts impact libido and physical comfort. Reducing misconceptions and promoting empathy are two benefits of knowing the biological underpinnings.

Seek Professional Advice: To address particular issues and investigate possible remedies, think about consulting healthcare practitioners or specialists in the field of sexual health.

9. Techniques for Positive Communication:

Expressing wishes: Promote candid discussion about preferences and wishes. Express your requirements in "I" phrases without blaming others.

Embracing Emotions: Respect each other's emotions without passing judgment. Acknowledge feelings and collaborate to come up with useful answers.

10. Give emotional connection top priority:

Strengthen Emotional Bonds: Since strong emotional bonds are the cornerstone of enduring closeness, emphasize strengthening them. To improve the emotional component of your relationship, talk about your hopes, worries, and thoughts.

Celebrate common Memories: By thinking back on and honoring common experiences, you may strengthen the link between people and create a feeling of community.

Encouraging intimacy and communication in the midst of menopause requires a dedication to understanding, adjusting, and placing equal emphasis on the mental and physical health of both partners. A robust and satisfying relationship is strengthened when both parties embrace this period of transformation with empathy and collaborative efforts. Couples may come out of the difficulties with a stronger bond and a fresh feeling of closeness.

- **Communicating with Loved Ones**

It is crucial to have effective communication throughout this stage to provide empathy, understanding, and support. These communication techniques might help you and your spouse or other family members or friends cope with menopause together:

1. Start Honest Discussions:

Establish Safe Spaces: Provide a setting where candid conversations are welcome. Make sure your loved one may express their sentiments without worrying about being judged.

Demonstrate Your Willingness to Listen: Inform them that you are ready to hear them out anytime they feel ready to speak.

2. Become Informed:

Study Menopause: Invest some time in learning about the mental and physical effects of menopause. Being aware of the changes makes it easier to provide knowledgeable assistance.

Read Aloud: To foster understanding, consider reading books or articles on menopause together.

3. Show Empathy for Shifts in Emotion:

Recognize Emotional Rollercoaster: Mood swings and emotional volatility are common side effects of menopause. Recognize that these shifts are an inherent part of the process and act with empathy and compassion.

Express Emotional Support: reassure them and let them know that you're ready to be there for them through good times and bad.

4. Promote Discussions About Symptoms:

Encourage your loved one to speak honestly about any physical or emotional issues they may be going through by encouraging open communication. Pay attention and give them credit for their experiences.

Pose Open-Ended Questions: To elicit more in-depth and insightful discussions, pose open-ended questions in instead of closed ones.

5. Take Part in Making Decisions:

Work Together to Find Solutions: Assist your loved one in making decisions about how to control their symptoms or adjust to changes in their lifestyle. Making decisions together fosters a feeling of collaboration.

Think About choices: When looking at possible interventions or solutions, be mindful of and respectful of their choices.

6. Provide Useful Assistance:

Help with Daily Tasks: Menopausal symptoms may be difficult to manage, so providing helpful assistance with everyday chores can have a big impact.

Communicate your availability to assist them with any needs they may have, including personal care and domestic duties.

7. Show Understanding and Patience:

Recognize the Transition: One of the biggest life transitions is going through menopause. Recognize that changes take time and exercise patience and understanding.

Express Commitment: Let them know that you are here to help them along the way and that you are in it for the long run.

8. Honour happy occasions:

Celebrate happy times and accomplishments that have to do with controlling menopausal symptoms or adjusting to changes.

Shared Joy: Reiterating a feeling of connection and understanding via sharing happy and humorous events.

9. Honour Individual Limitations:

Realize the Need for Space: Appreciate the value of your own space and self-care. Give them the freedom to put their own needs first and respect their limits.

Encourage Open Communication Regarding Limits: To promote mutual understanding, promote open communication regarding personal needs and limits.

10. Seek Expert Advice in Concert:

Examine Therapeutic help: If necessary, think about going together to acquire therapeutic help. Expert advice may encourage honest dialogue and provide resources for overcoming obstacles.

Togetherness in Therapy: Having therapy sessions together fosters a cooperative mindset in recognizing and resolving the effects of menopause on relationships.

11. Show your affection and love:

Verbal Affirmations: Use spoken affirmations to show your love and devotion. Tell your loved one how much you value their health and well-being.

Physical Touch: To strengthen a feeling of connection, provide physical comfort by giving hugs or other little gestures.

12. Preserve Your Sense of Humour:

Laugh Together: Look for opportunities to laugh together. Humor is a great tool for overcoming obstacles and forging strong bonds with others. Lighten the Mood: Whenever appropriate, inject humor into conversations to make them more fun and less serious.

Menopause-related effective communication requires constant attempts to comprehend, empathize with, and assist your loved one. You may both feel heard and supported as you traverse this transitional period together if you approach the trip with patience, openness, and a shared commitment to each other's well-being.

• Building a Support Network

It's important to surround oneself with compassionate and understanding people who can provide support, direction, and company as a person going through menopause. Here are some tips for creating a strong support system throughout menopause:

1. Being Honest with Those You Love:

Talk About Your Experience: Have honest discussions about your menopausal experience with your spouse, family, and close friends. Assist them in understanding your needs, struggles, and experiences.

Set Clear Expectations: Let someone know exactly what sort of help you may need, including emotional support, help with everyday chores, or just someone to listen.

2. Establish Contact with Menopausal People:

Join Support Groups: Look for menopausal support groups in your area or online where people can relate to one another and exchange stories.

Attend seminars or activities: Take part in menopause-related seminars or activities. This offers a chance to interact with those going through comparable situations.

3. Interact with Medical Experts:

Consult Healthcare Providers: Form close relationships with medical experts who specialize in menopause and women's health. Personalized guidance and medical assistance are guaranteed when you have regular check-ups and consultations.

Never be afraid to clarify anything you don't understand about any part of menopause by asking questions. A knowledgeable medical staff may be a great asset to your support system.

4. Promote Family Engagement:

Educate Family Members: Give your family information on menopause so they can comprehend the possible emotional and physical changes you may be going through.

Involve Family in Self-Care: To foster a supportive and active atmosphere, invite family members to join you in self-care activities.

5. Ask Your Friends for Help:

Talk to friends about your menopausal journey by sharing your experiences. Friends may give insightful stories or important ideas, and they can also offer sympathetic understanding.

Arrange events Together: Take part in social events that encourage unwinding and having fun, strengthening your bonds with pals.

6. Provide Support in the Workplace:

Talk to Coworkers: To promote understanding in the workplace, feel free to talk to managers or other coworkers about menopause.

Request Accommodations if Needed: To guarantee a supportive work environment, if menopausal symptoms interfere with your employment, think about seeking accommodations or modifications.

7. Participate in Online Groups:

Investigate Online Forums: Take part in online forums or groups where people discuss their menopausal experiences. This online community may foster a feeling of belonging and serve as a forum for advice-sharing.

8. Establish Contact with Mental Health Experts:

Because menopause might affect mental health, think about therapy. If necessary, look into counseling or therapy alternatives with mental health specialists who specialize in women's health.

Prioritise Emotional Well-Being: During this time, acknowledge the significance of your mental and emotional health and, if needed, seek professional assistance.

9. Go to Educational Events:

Take Part in Seminars or Webinars: Attend educational menopausal events to learn more about the topic and make connections with professionals.

Opportunities for Networking: Take advantage of these gatherings to meet others going through comparable situations and form relationships.

10. Invite your partners to the event:

Invite Partners to Activities: Try to get your spouse to come along to support group meetings or educational activities. This may improve their comprehension and fortify your network of support.

11. Make self-care a priority:

Choose Self-Care Activities: Look into self-care activities that you find meaningful and give them top priority in your daily schedule.

Express Your Requirements: Make sure your support system is aware of your requirements for self-care so they can help you to facilitate these routines.

12. Be Willing to Make New Friends:

Embrace New Connections: Menopause may be a chance to meet new people who are aware of and supportive of this period of life.

Network Within Communities: To increase the size of your support system, get in touch with community centers, wellness groups, or women's health organizations.

During menopause, proactive communication, asking loved ones for understanding, and interacting with a variety of resources are all important components of developing a solid support system. Having a diverse support network throughout this life-changing stage improves your general well-being in addition to assisting you in overcoming obstacles.

Chapter 7

Menopause and Beyond

A new act that goes much beyond hormonal fluctuations and reproductive changes starts as the menopausal era comes to an end. This stage, appropriately named "Menopause and Beyond," is characterized by a journey of deep self-realization, individual empowerment, and a reinterpretation of what it means to be in good health. The early years after menopause are a time of emancipation. Women feel liberated when their monthly periods stop, freeing them from the biological patterns that traditionally dictated their existence. As the hormones settle into a harmonic tune, a new balance arises, providing the groundwork for delving into more profound aspects of oneself.

Living after menopause is like entering a broad field of self-awareness. Hormonal fluctuations whirlwind slowly fade, exposing the features of inner strength that may have escaped attention during the turbulent menopausal years. This power turns into a driving force that helps people live a life that is purposefully molded by their own goals and objectives.

This postmenopausal chapter emphasizes accepting oneself. The stories that society taught about youth and fertility start to fade. After emerging from the menopausal cocoon, women have a deep appreciation for the beauty that accompanies aging. Not flaws, but marks of a life well lived, wrinkles bear witness to tenacity, humor, and the passing of time with every line.

The emotional terrain becomes more serene. The choppy waves of menopausal feelings give way to a serene lake of introspection. Intimate and platonic relationships alike gain from this improved emotional balance. As people develop genuine, caring, and satisfying relationships, their bonds get stronger because they are more aware of their emotional needs. Life beyond menopause is a tribute to overall health. Instead of being the pursuit of goals outside oneself, physical health becomes a celebration of the body's eternal life. A life that is not merely lived but lived vibrantly is facilitated by the daily rituals of exercise, nourishing food, and mindfulness practices.

Once a representation of loss, the empty nest becomes a place of rediscovery. Women find themselves at the cusp of uncharted territory as their children carve out their own pathways. Rekindled interests, hobbies, and long-forgotten goals are followed with a vigor that only comes with age and knowledge.

Women are more confidently embracing leadership responsibilities in the workplace. Their extensive experience and acquired knowledge over the years enable them to act as change agents, making distinctive contributions to their communities and businesses. Being a grandmother brings happiness and knowledge. The affection and care that they used to provide to their own children now easily trickle down to the next generation. Women become storytellers when they become grandparents, imparting life lessons learned from navigating the ups and downs.

Life after menopause is a colorful encore rather than a conclusion. It's a journey where women bravely negotiate the difficulties of the world with the knowledge gained from their experiences. Every day is welcomed with appreciation, and every obstacle is faced with the fortitude that comes from having lived a life well lived.

These ladies go into the dark with confidence, their hearts full of thankfulness and their spirits ready for the dawn of every new day, as the sun sets on each new one. "Menopause and Beyond" is more than simply a stage; it's a tribute to the eternal beauty, wisdom, and power that accompany a woman's life journey.

Conclusion

- **Empowering Women in Their Menopausal Journey**

In summary, the menopausal experience is a life-changing event that merits acknowledgment, joy, and most importantly, empowerment. Encouraging women to embrace this era with grace and fortitude is crucial as they negotiate the difficult landscape of hormonal shifts, bodily changes, and emotional upheavals.

Recognizing the strength inherent in this life-changing experience is the first step towards empowering women through menopause. Instead of being a tale of decline, the menopause story is one of women's resiliency, as they face changes with a toughness that has been built over years of varied experiences. Acknowledging and appreciating this strength turns into a cornerstone of empowerment.

Awareness and education are yet another essential component of empowerment. We empower women to make educated choices by arming them with full information on menopause, including its physiological features and associated emotional effects. Comprehending the subtleties of menopause fosters a feeling of mastery and autonomy for an individual's own welfare.

One cannot exaggerate the importance of support and community. An environment of support is created when women are connected via networks where they may exchange experiences, provide guidance, and listen with empathy. The notion that women are not alone in their menopausal journey is strengthened by the inspiration and support this group provides.

Empowerment begins with promoting open communication in families and the workplace. We dispel gender stereotypes around menopause by creating spaces where women feel free to communicate their needs and difficulties. This transparency makes it easier to comprehend, support, and break down long-standing taboos.

In the empowerment story, holistic well-being—which includes mental, emotional, and physical health—becomes central. Encouraging mindfulness, a healthy lifestyle, and self-care techniques all support a woman's general well-being both during and after menopause.

Additionally, professional empowerment is quite important. Women may succeed in their professions provided their needs are met and their contributions to the workforce at this time of life are acknowledged. Women who are empowered at work not only support their own development but also the overall health of their companies.

Menopause is a special thread in the vast tapestry of life that ties a woman's perseverance, power, and knowledge into her identity. It's a progression towards a more powerful, real self, not a waning of energy.

It is our social responsibility to encourage, inspire, and celebrate women as they go through menopause. We contribute to a narrative that empowers women not just during menopause but throughout their whole lives by creating places that recognize and honor the strength and wisdom earned during this era of life. It is a group celebration of the resilient spirit of women, honoring the strength, intelligence, and beauty present at each stage of their journey.

THANK YOU FOR CHOOSING US.

We Appreciate Your Kind Support And We Hope You Got Something Out Of It.

If You Enjoy This Book, It Will Be Great To Leave a **Review On Amazon** . It Means a Lot To Us.